Birth Yoga
Mother's Guide

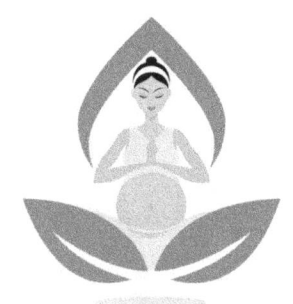

Birth Yoga
Mother's Guide

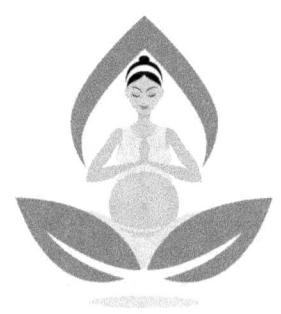

Donyale Abe

I dedicate this book to women everywhere

You're powerful

You're strong

You can

You are

You will

Namaste

This is my guide

_____

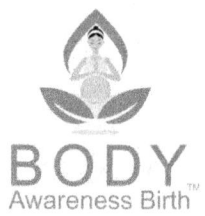

Table of Contents

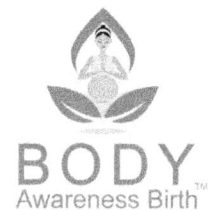

About

This booklet is written to accompany Body Awareness Birth™ Yoga classes.

In *Birth Yoga Mother's Guide* we have combined our three best selling booklets:

> The Transformation of Pregnancy
>
> The Journey to Birth My Baby
>
> Birth Hopes and Dreams

Feel free to use this guide without attending classes, however you will gain more if you are able to attend a birth yoga class. If there are not any in your area search for a prenatal yoga class.

We share this guide to help you explore the wonderment of pregnancy, face the challenge of labor and discover the power of birth.

In your birth yoga class your teacher will guide you through a brief reflective lesson. You will then receive a suggested birth yoga pose that you can do on your own.

Please bring your booklet to class each week.

The Transformation of Pregnancy

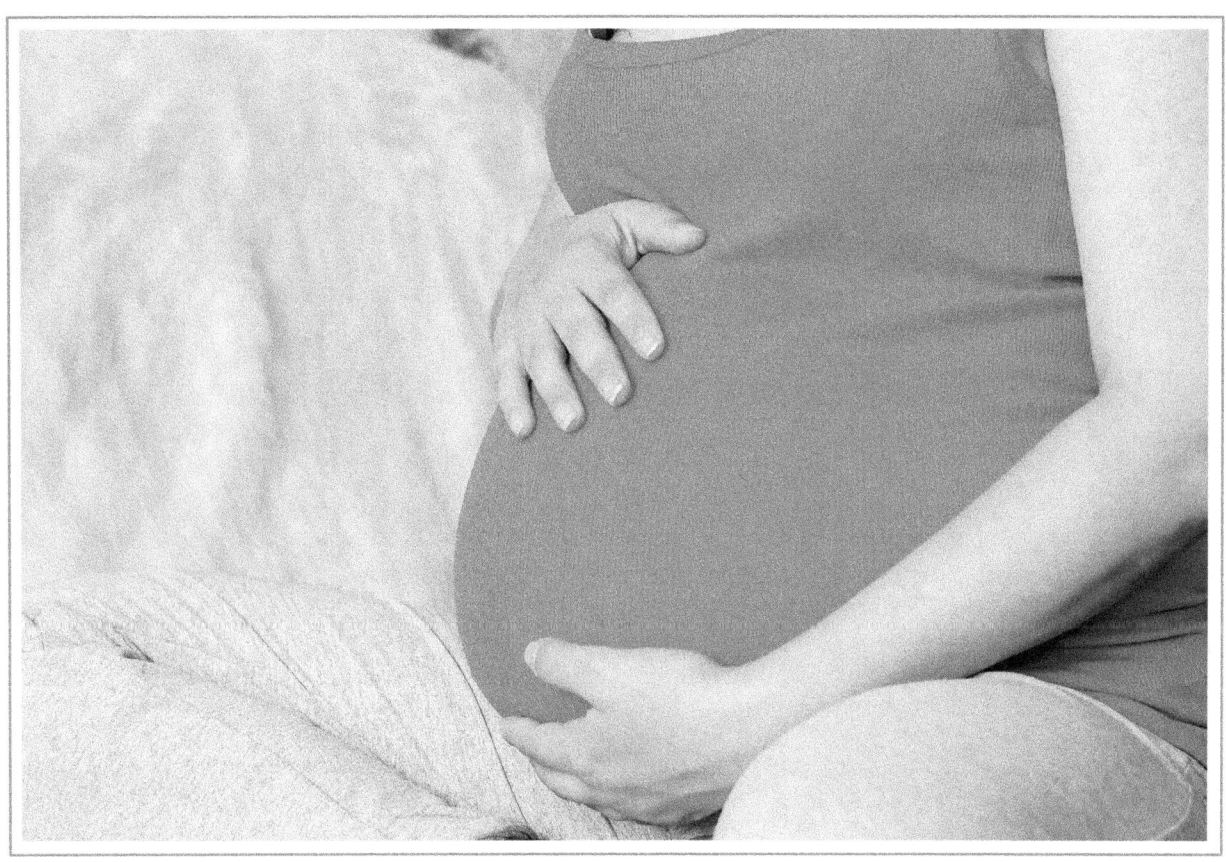

The Transformation of Pregnancy © 2014 by Donyale Abe

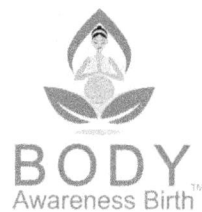

Birth Yoga™

Thank you for allowing us to share in your journey of pregnancy, birth, and motherhood.

How has your experience been so far? _____

_____

_____

It is our intention that you feel supported through this experience, as you participate in Body Awareness Birth Yoga classes or B.A.B.Y. classes.

Our sessions are designed to build

Community

Knowledge

Inner Strength

Body Awareness

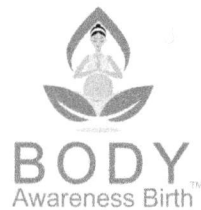

Tuning-In

We will take time each class to practice being present in the moment. Not to dwell on what happened during your week, day, or the hour before you came to BABY class, but to let everything go. Be present in this moment. The ability to be present will help you during labor and serve to guide you through motherhood.

Write down one emotion you feel in this moment?

_____

If it is positive hold on to it and if it is not positive release it. Embrace this moment.

You and your baby are the focus of our sessions. Birth yoga class is a safe space created for you to let go, embrace yourself, connect to your baby and just be.

You may find in just being that you are filled with hopes and dreams. Your self awareness, inner knowledge, and determination may increase.

Write down one thing you can do to pamper yourself this week?
(Even if it's quick i.e. soak your feet.)

_____

_____

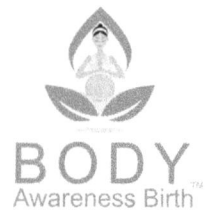

Affirmations

Words are powerful tools

A key component of our Body Awareness Birth Yoga classes is affirmation. Affirmations are positive and praising words to focus our minds upon. Affirmations are a reservoir of all that you need, when you are in need.

Notice what non-positive words or messages you hear each day.

Replace them with an affirmation. Ask those close to you to be affirming.

Tell them your affirmation so they can say it to you.

Write down your affirmations

I am _____

Other Affirmations _____

_____

_____

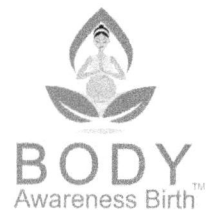

Body Awareness

Pregnant women often feel many sensations they have never experienced before. The pregnant body is equipped to recognize if it likes or dislikes a sensation.

While the body is automated and functions independently to create a baby, the mind works slowly to process what is going on.

The body is always right. It signals our mind all day long with messages of how we truly are.

What is your body telling you? _____

Have you missed any key signals?

Eating   Discomfort

Sleeping   Going to restroom

Illness

Trusting your body

Listen to your body. Become aware of its signals. Take one moment each day to jot down what your body is telling you.

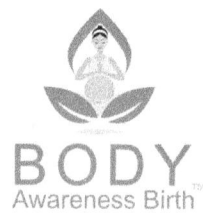
On your own

Sit in easy pose. Connect to your breath.

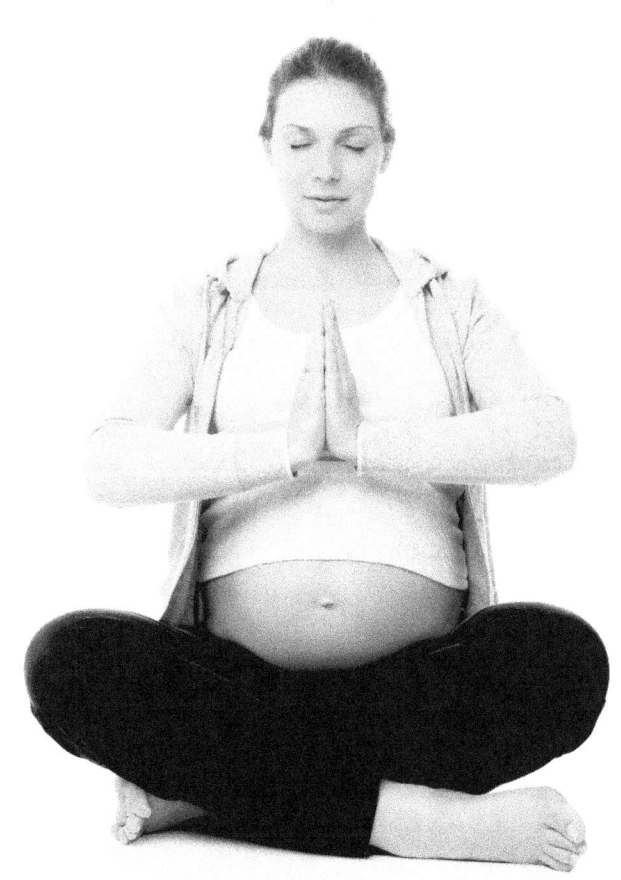

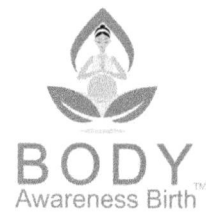
Changing You

What's happening

So a baby is growing and growing inside your uterus.

How is the power of creating another human changing you? _____

_____

A pregnant woman has double the blood volume she normally would to reproduce cells and grow nutrients to produce a healthy baby.

You are producing relaxin a hormone that allows your bones to stretch and shift creating space for your baby to pass through your pelvic bones and out the birth canal.

Pregnant women have increased sensory awareness. This is nature's way to protect the very young from harm.

Senses

Touch	Sight
Taste	Hear
Smell	Intuition

What is your intuition or sixth sense telling you?

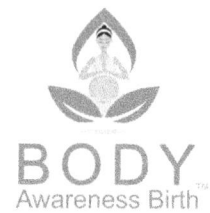

On your own

Take time for yourself. Enjoy the moment.

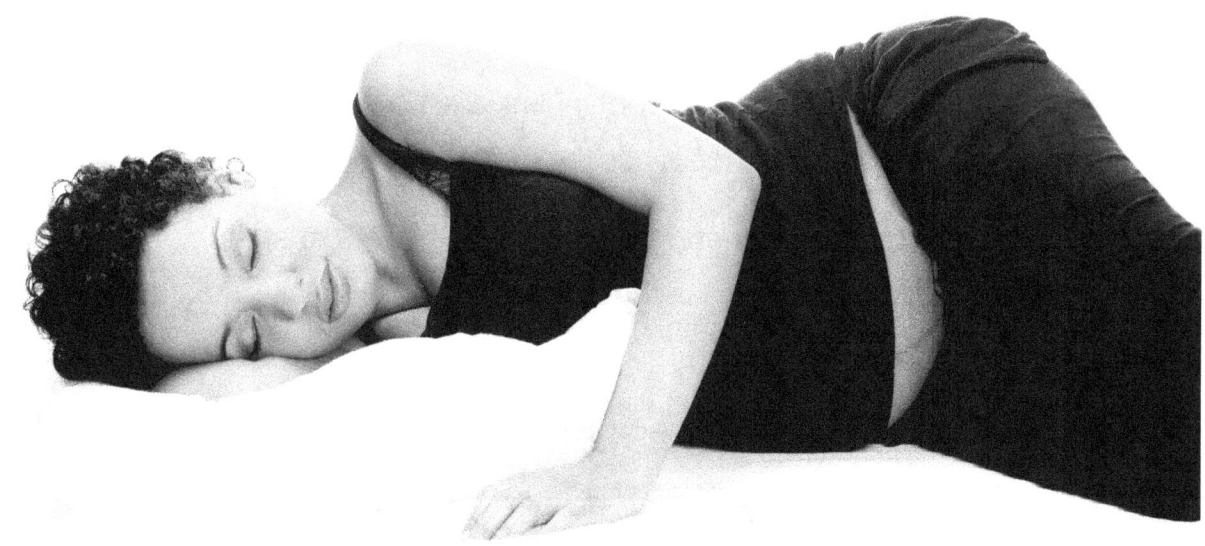

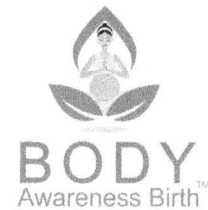

More Than One

Understanding that

Inside your body for a short while are two minds and two hearts. If you are having multiple babies even more...

How do you feel about being more than one? _____

_____

_____

Interesting Information

A healthy, full term pregnancy lasts from 37 to 42 weeks. Due dates are correct only 3% of the time.

Babies inside the womb like to share your life. Have you noticed your baby likes music? They love voices. Babies like when you eat. They like it when you talk to them.

Write a card or letter to your baby

If you like bring to the next class to share.

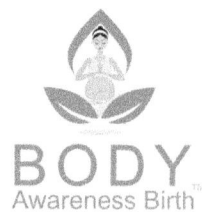

On your own

Connect to your baby. Connect to your breath.

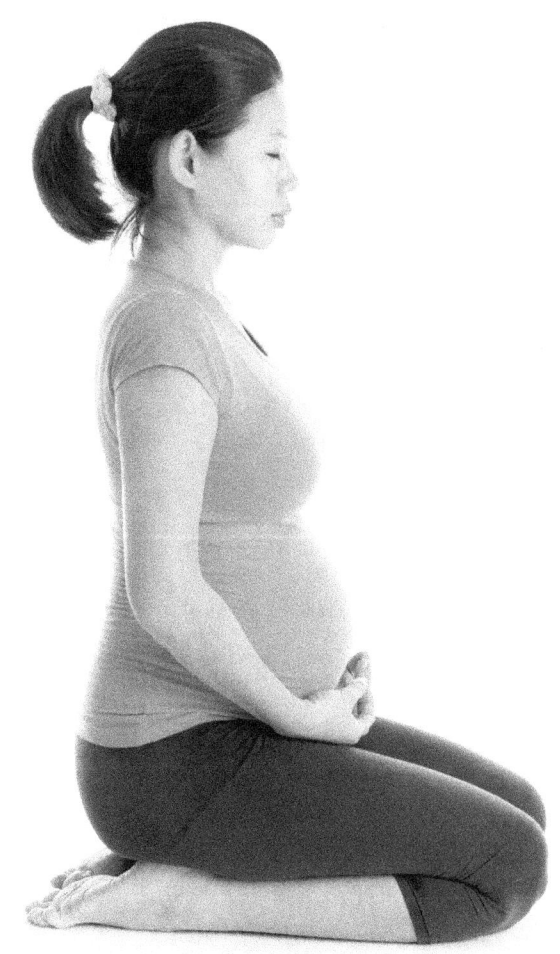

The Journey to Birth My Baby

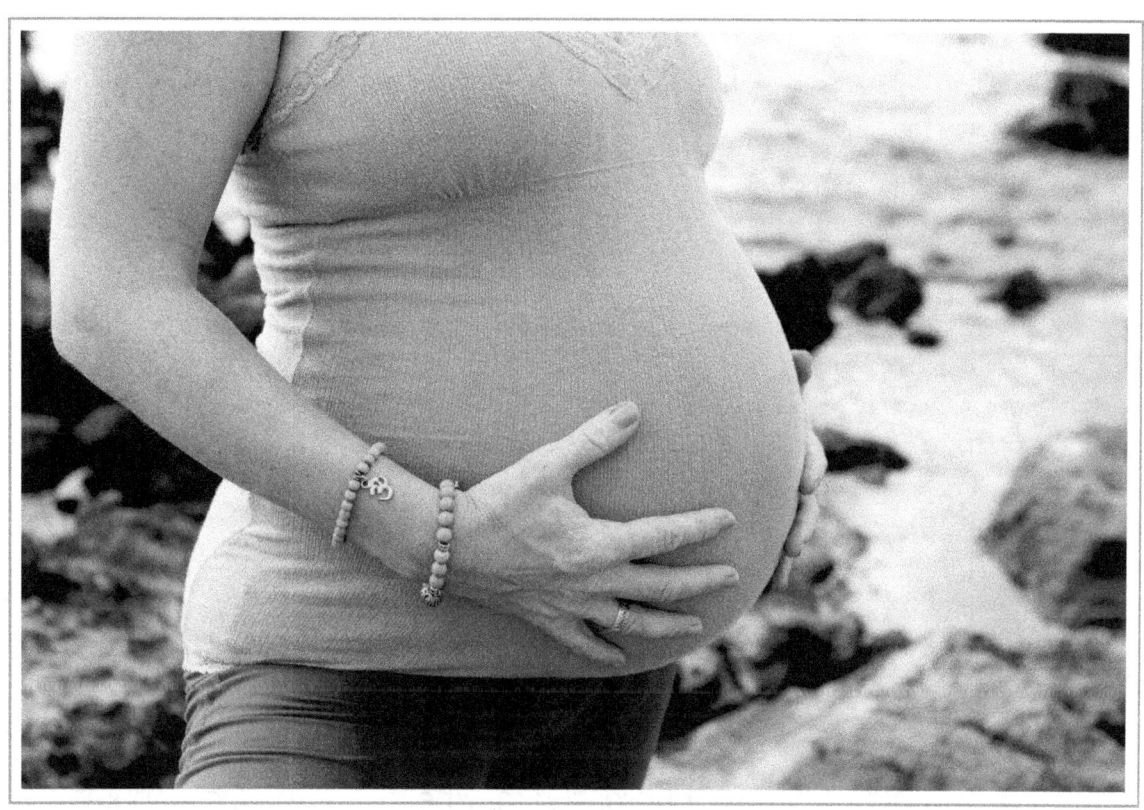

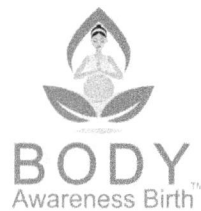

Your Body

Accomplishes amazing things

A woman's body grows and nurtures her baby as she goes about day to day activities. Eyelashes, eyebrows, and eyes are formed. The complex brain develops. Tiny fingers and toes start to wiggle.

Within your body lies the extraordinary power that is creating your baby and will guide you through birth.

Reflect upon the power of your body

Your body creates relaxin, a hormone that loosens your hips and ligaments creating space for your baby to pass through your pelvic bones for birth.

Your body creates oxytocin a hormone that causes your uterus to contract eventually resulting in the birth of your baby.

Your uterus normally the size of your fist expands and nurtures your baby helping it grow. When in pain your body makes endorphins similar to the narcotic morphine helping you cope with the intensity of birth. There's much more...

Write down what amazes you about your body

_____

_____

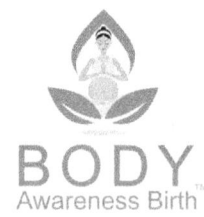

On your own

Come into child's pose. Connect to your breath.

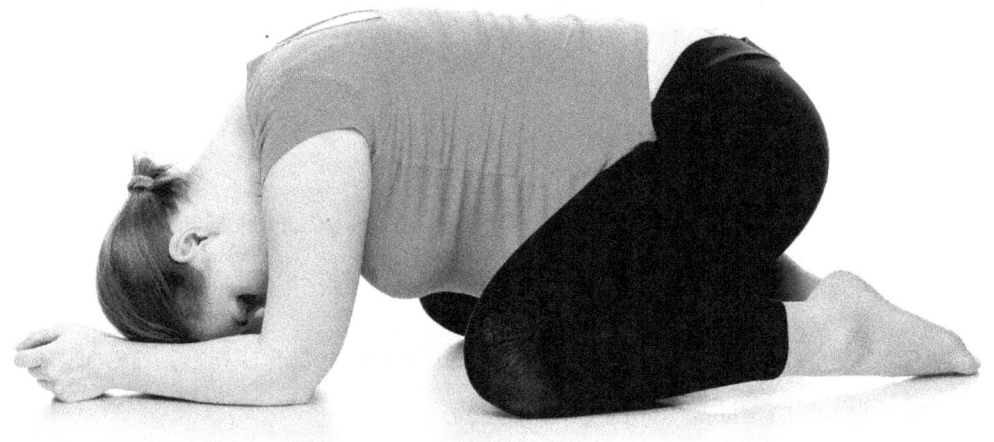

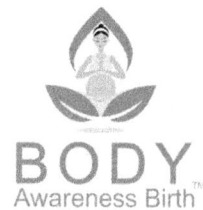

Your Baby

Is so incredible

No closer connection exists between humans than being in the womb. Inside your safe womb your baby is getting to know you. They know your smell, your rhythms, your voice, your language, and more.

And you know your baby. Already you know their patterns. You can sense their favorite spot inside of you. You know when they have hiccups. You know what they favor when you play music or eat food.

You and your baby are a team. You need each other. You give strength to each other. Your baby knows when to be born. In your womb when full development is reached your baby will secrete a hormone initiating your body to start the labor process.

Imagine those first moments gazing at your baby in your arms

Write what words you might speak to your baby at birth

_____

_____

_____

Take this moment to connect to your baby. Share your heart.

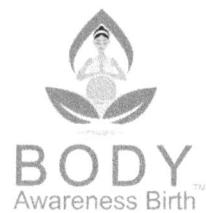

On your own

Get on your hands and knees. Raise your back up like a cat. Feel your baby shift.

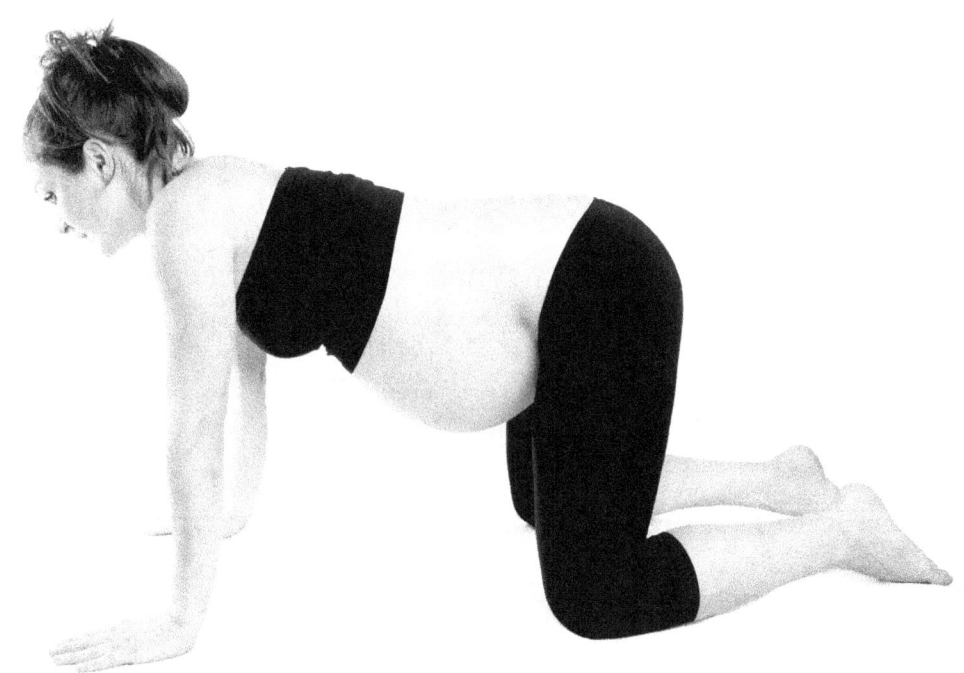

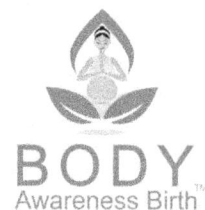

Your Birth

A rite of passage

Birth is so personal. It is your journey. No one can take it for you. Birth is as old as time. Most of the women that have existed on the planet we call earth have given birth successfully, else where would humans be? However to fear birth is normal.

What fears or concerns do you have?

_____

_____

Your mind and heart play an important role in giving birth. Filling your inner self with affirming and positive thoughts, as well as having knowledge about the process of birth will help squelch any fears and empower you through birth.

What do you personally need to give birth?

_____

_____

_____

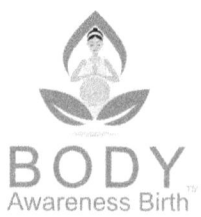

On your own

Sit in easy pose. Bring your palms together. Connect to your breath and baby.

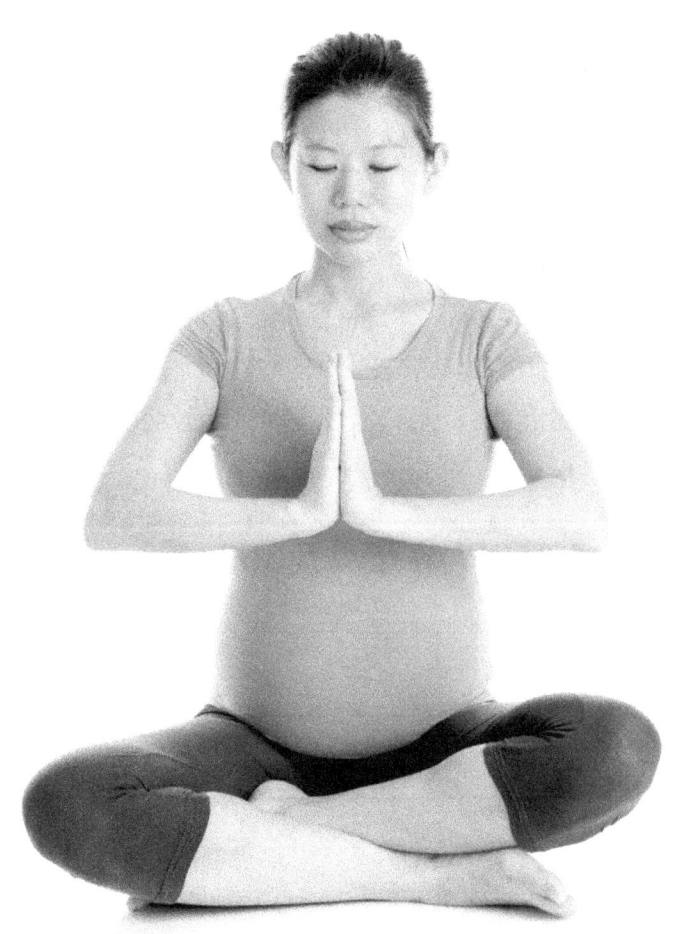

Birth Hopes and Dreams

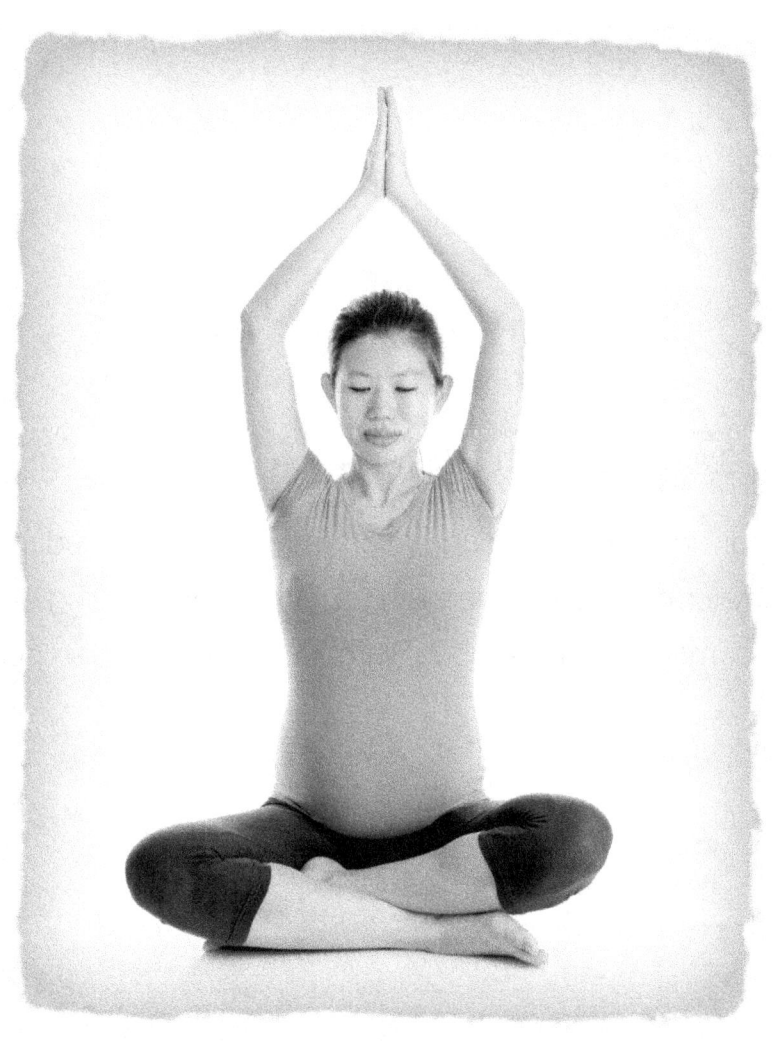

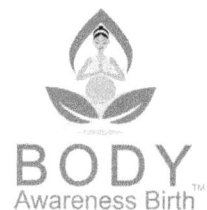

Hopes

Bring change

Hope is that longing and knowing that something good is on the way. Your baby.

Babies have a funny way of making us hope.

You hope your baby will be healthy. You hope for a boy. You hope for a girl. You hope your baby will be early. You hope your labor will be quick.

Hope assures you that even when things get challenging that all will turn out well. Hope will brighten your day! Your hopes influence your baby to be. There's nothing that you can't hope for...

Write down your personal hopes

_____

_____

_____

_____

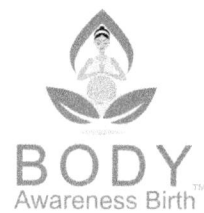
On your own

Come into easy pose. Connect to your breath.

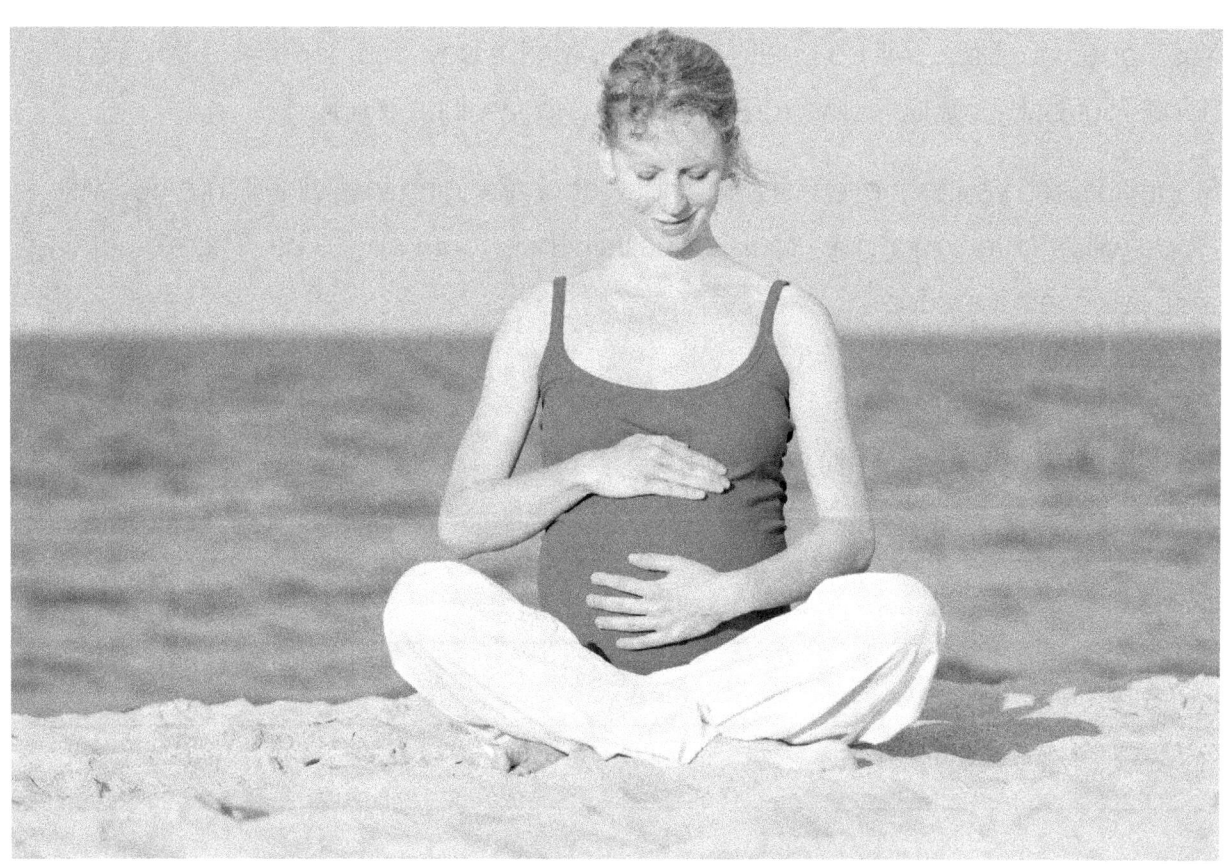

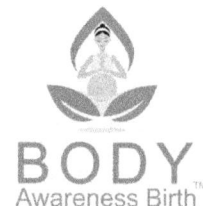

BODY
Awareness Birth™

Dreams

Are vivid during pregnancy

Pregnant women can dream in technicolor. It is common to have intense, elaborate, overwhelming dreams during your time of pregnancy.

You may dream as you sleep or you may just dream in your heart, or in your thoughts.

Your dreams may just be a knowingness of what is to come.

In a mother's dreams everything is possible.

Reflect on your dreams as you prepare for labor and birth

Think about your dream birth. Consider the dreams you have for your baby and for your new family. Each child born is a new dream, a new beginning. Don't let your dreams be squelched. Hold them close. Believe in them.

Jot down a few of your dreams

_____

_____

_____

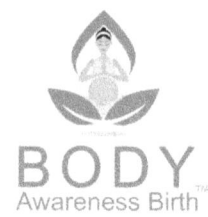

On your own

Sit in the floor with the soles of your feet touching. Try a gentle butterfly.

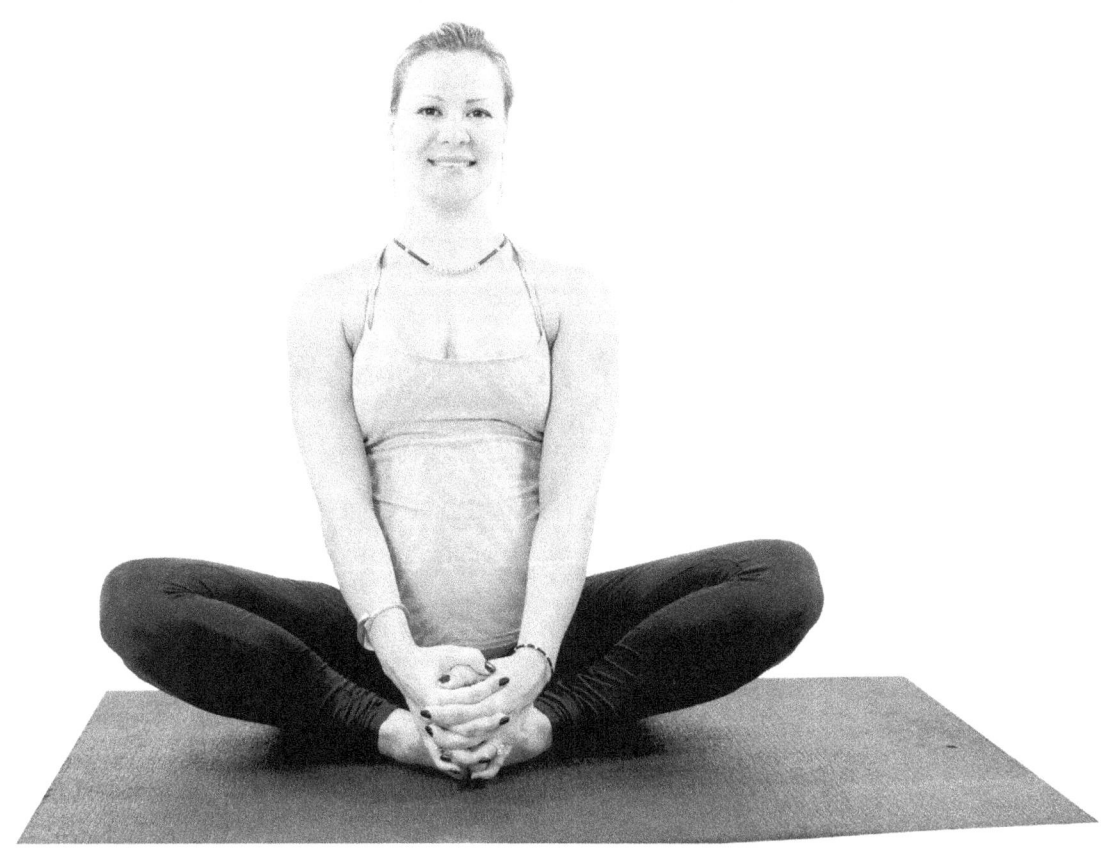

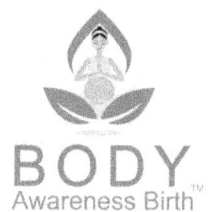

Knowledge

Seek to know as much as possible

You are ready with your hopes and dreams so...Are you ready for whatever may come your way during the process of pregnancy, labor, birth, and motherhood. There is a lot to it.

Knowledge is power. So ask as many questions as you can. Your doctor, midwife, and other care providers should be able to explain things to you. Don't feel pressured to make decisions.

Even in the throes of labor you should feel *right* with all procedures and understand what is happening. If your instinct tells you something...listen!

And don't be afraid to speak up. One way to approach a conversation with your doctor is to ask what are the benefits, risks, and alternatives to any procedure they suggest.

Knowledge Check-In

Circle the areas you need to know more about

Medications	Breastfeeding
Baby care	Labor Process
Breathing & Relaxation Techniques	Water Birth
Doulas	Postpartum Depression
Midwifery Care	Interventions i.e. breaking waters

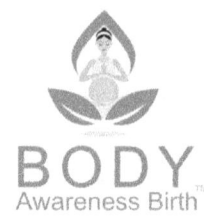
On your own

Sit on your heals. Reach your palms behind you for a gentle stretch.

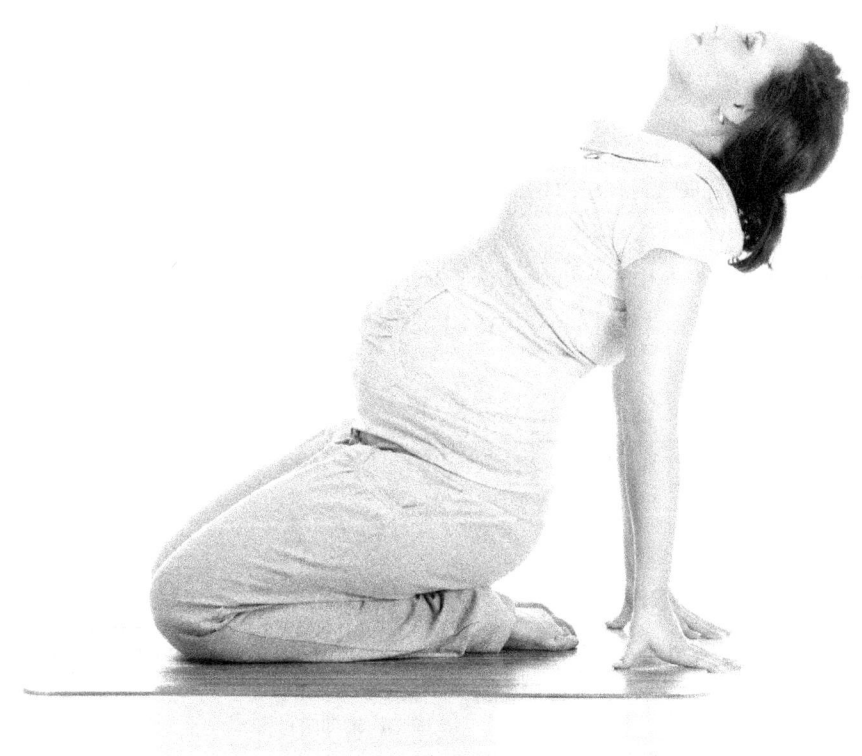

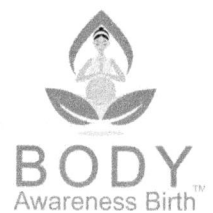

Birth Yoga Booklet Series

The Transformation of Pregnancy

The Journey to Birth My Baby

Birth Hopes and Dreams

Facilitating Birth Yoga

Booklets can be ordered

thechildbirthprofession.com/birthyoga

JOIN OUR BIRTH YOGA TEACHER TRAINING WORKSHOPS

Learn to empower pregnant women and to facilitate body awareness birth yoga sessions.

Website: thechildbirthprofession.com/birthyoga

Email: birtheducators@gmail.com

Phone: 916-525-7596

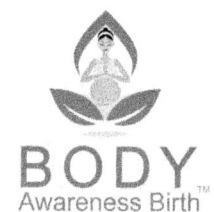